Unveiling the Ancient Secret to Glowing Skin:

A Bison Tallow Revolution

Johnny D. Mulder

Imagine a time before chemical concoctions lined bathroom shelves. People relied on the wisdom of nature, using what the earth provided to nourish and protect their skin. **"The Bison Tallow Beauty Revolution"** embarks on an adventure to rediscover this forgotten secret: the potent power of bison tallow.

This isn't just another skincare guide; it's a call to arms. It's an invitation to shed the synthetic shackles and embrace a **renaissance of natural beauty**.

Picture this: Our ancestors, braving the elements on the American plains, their skin thriving thanks to a remarkable substance – bison tallow. This age-old remedy, cast aside in the 20th century's rush for artificial alternatives, is poised for a grand comeback.

Why? Because the 21st century craves **sustainable solutions**. Bison tallow offers unparalleled benefits with its unique blend of fatty acids and vitamins. Forget harsh chemicals; this natural wonder promises to **hydrate, revitalize, and repair your skin**.

This book shatters the myths surrounding animal fats in skincare. We'll delve into the **science, expert insights, and historical context**, revealing how bison

Chapter 1:

From Ancient Ritual to Modern Marvel: The Bison Tallow Revival

Imagine a time before fancy labels and chemical concoctions. Imagine Native American tribes braving the harsh elements, their skin remarkably smooth and protected. Their secret? A gift from the mighty bison – its tallow.

This chapter embarks on a captivating journey, tracing the path of bison tallow from **ancient wisdom to a modern revolution** in the world of cosmetics.

Picture this: Vast herds of bison thundered across the North American plains. These majestic creatures weren't just a source of food and shelter; they were the key to radiant skin. Native Americans, with their deep respect for nature, discovered the **potent properties of bison tallow**.

Rich in fatty acids that mimic human skin, this natural wonder offered superior protection and hydration. It wasn't just a basic moisturizer; it formed the base for healing salves and ointments, a testament to their profound understanding of nature's bounty.

However, as European settlers encroached westward, the bison population dwindled. With them, the knowledge of their diverse uses, including this **forgotten beauty secret**, started to fade.

Fast forward to the 20th century. Synthetic ingredients took center stage, pushing natural alternatives like bison tallow to the sidelines.

But the tide is turning. The 21st century is witnessing a **resurgence of natural beauty solutions**. Consumers are becoming increasingly conscious of the impact of harsh chemicals, seeking alternatives that are **sustainable and kind to their skin**.

Enter Bison Tallow, back in the spotlight. **Minimally processed and remarkably compatible with human skin**, it's become a star ingredient in the natural beauty movement.

This chapter takes you on a captivating voyage. We'll explore:

- **The ancient legacy:** How Native Americans harnessed the power of bison tallow.

- **A forgotten treasure:** The decline of bison and the fading knowledge of its uses.
- **The modern revival:** Why bison tallow is experiencing a remarkable comeback.
- **Science meets nature:** Unveiling the science behind bison tallow's remarkable skin benefits.
- **The new generation:** Highlighting the stories of modern artisans and entrepreneurs who are rediscovering this ancient beauty secret.

Join us as we delve into the fascinating world of bison tallow, a testament to the enduring power of nature's wisdom and a symbol of a new era in sustainable and effective skincare.

Chapter 2:
Cracking the Code: Bison Tallow's Skin—Loving Science

Remember that time your grandma used a secret salve to soothe your sunburn? Turns out, there might be some truth to those old-fashioned remedies. This chapter dives into the fascinating science behind Bison Tallow, the **rising star of natural skincare**.

Imagine this: Picture your skin as a complex ecosystem protected by a natural oil barrier. Bison tallow, with its unique blend of fatty acids, **mimics this barrier almost perfectly**. It's like a key fitting seamlessly into a lock. This allows for **deeper, non-greasy moisturization**, unlike harsh chemicals that can clog pores and disrupt your skin's natural balance.

But bison tallow does more than just hydrate. It's a **multitasking marvel**.

- **Feeling the heat?** Bison tallow's **anti-inflammatory properties** can calm irritated skin, a welcome relief for those prone to redness or flare-ups.
- **Think of it as a tiny vitamin factory.** Bison tallow is packed with vitamins A, D,

E, and K. Vitamin A helps your skin **regenerate**, D keeps it **healthy**, E acts as a powerful **antioxidant** shield, and K plays a vital role in **healing and elasticity**.

The good news? Bison tallow is suitable for almost everyone.

- **Sensitive skin?** Its **antibacterial properties** can help maintain a balanced microbiome, preventing breakouts.
- **Dry or damaged skin?** Bison tallow provides essential fatty acids to **repair the barrier**, locking in moisture and protecting you from environmental aggressors.

This chapter isn't just about scientific jargon. We'll also hear real stories: **people just like you sharing their experiences** with this natural wonder. From overcoming chronic dryness to achieving a radiant glow, these **personal testimonies** showcase the transformative power of bison tallow.

Get ready to **unwrap the science behind this age-old secret** and discover why bison tallow is taking the natural beauty world by storm. Through a blend of **engaging storytelling and insightful**

facts, we'll unveil the full potential of this remarkable ingredient, proving that sometimes, grandma's wisdom might just be the key to healthy, glowing skin.

Chapter 3:
Beauty with a Conscience: The Sustainable Story of Bison Tallow

Picture this: lush green plains teeming with bison, these majestic creatures roaming free. But here's the surprising part: their role goes beyond simply providing delicious meat. Bison tallow, a natural byproduct, is making waves in the beauty world for its effectiveness and its **sustainable and ethical story**.

This chapter dives into the heart of what makes bison tallow a **beacon of hope** for eco-conscious consumers.

Remember the near-extinction of the bison? Thankfully, thanks to dedicated conservation efforts, these giants are back. But their story goes beyond survival. Today, bison are raised with a purpose – to **restore the very land they graze on**.

Imagine vast fields mimicking the natural movements of wild herds. This **rotational grazing** isn't just good for the bison; it **revitalizes the soil and the entire ecosystem**.

Ethical sourcing is key. We'll meet passionate farmers who prioritize the **well-being of their animals and the health of the land**. These heroes operate under **regenerative agriculture principles**, promoting biodiversity, improving water cycles, and even helping capture carbon from the atmosphere.

By choosing bison tallow from such sources, you're not just treating your skin; you're **contributing to a positive environmental impact**.

Here's the beauty of it all: Since tallow is a byproduct of the meat industry, it **minimizes waste**. It's a philosophy of **respect and responsibility**, ensuring nothing goes to waste. This aligns perfectly with the **circular economy**, where every part of the bison is valued.

Get ready to be inspired. We'll hear from **farmers, conservationists, and even beauty experts**. They'll share the challenges and triumphs of bringing this **ancient ingredient** into the modern world, proving that **beauty can truly go hand-in-hand with sustainability**.

This chapter is about more than skincare; it's about making informed choices that benefit our appearance and the planet we call home.

Chapter 4:

DIY Bison Tallow Magic: Whip Up Your Own Skincare Wonders

Imagine this: shelves overflowing with fancy creams and potions, yet your skin still feels...lackluster. What if the answer lies not in mass-produced products but in your own hands? This chapter empowers you to unleash your inner alchemist and craft **powerful, personalized skincare** using the magic of bison tallow.

Why DIY? It's not just about the satisfaction of creating something yourself. It's about **knowing exactly what you're putting on your skin**. Bison tallow, with its rich heritage and a treasure trove of benefits, becomes the hero ingredient in your DIY journey.

Ready to get started? The first step is sourcing high-quality bison tallow. Remember the ethical sourcing practices discussed in Chapter 3. Look for brands that prioritize **happy, healthy animals and a thriving planet**.

Once you have your golden ticket, the possibilities are endless! We'll explore

simple recipes to get you started, from lip balms that pamper your pout to luxurious moisturizers and soothing salves.

Cracked lips got you down? Our **easy lip balm recipe** combines the magic of bison tallow with beeswax and coconut oil. Add a dash of your favorite essential oil for a delightful scent and a touch of extra TLC.

Dry, flaky skin? This **deeply hydrating moisturizer** is your new best friend. We'll show you how to blend bison tallow with shea butter, jojoba oil, and aloe vera gel for a **silky smooth** finish that lasts.

Skin feeling a bit worse for wear? Bison tallow's **anti-inflammatory properties** come to the rescue in this **healing salve**. We'll guide you through melting tallow with an herb-infused carrier oil (think calendula or chamomile for extra goodness). A touch of beeswax for thickness and vitamin E oil for an extra boost, and voila! Your skin will thank you for the **soothing relief**.

Remember, these are just the stepping stones! As you gain confidence, experiment with different ingredients and ratios. This is your chance to create **unique products** that perfectly address your skin's needs and preferences.

Embrace the **DIY spirit** and embark on a journey towards a more **sustainable and conscious beauty routine**. Your skin will radiate, and you'll have the satisfaction of knowing you created something special just for you.

Chapter 5:

From Kitchen Counter to Cosmetic Counter: Building Your Bison Tallow Empire

Ever dreamt of transforming your DIY passion into a full-blown skincare brand? This chapter equips you to take the leap and **build your own bison tallow empire**. But remember, this isn't just about mixing ingredients in your kitchen anymore.

We'll guide you through the exciting yet intricate process of **creating advanced, effective, and safe skincare products** using bison tallow as your star ingredient.

First things first: Not everyone has the same skin. Understanding **different skin types and their needs** is crucial. Dryness, aging, sensitivity – your bison tallow creations need to be tailored to combat these concerns.

The good news? Bison Tallow is a **skincare chameleon**. Because it closely mimics our natural oils, it blends beautifully with other active ingredients. This allows you to create a diverse range of products that target specific issues, from combating wrinkles to calming breakouts.

But crafting these wonders requires a touch of **science along with the art**. Imagine yourself as a cosmetic chemist, understanding how emulsions work, how to choose the proper preservatives and the importance of maintaining the perfect pH balance. Remember, a stable product is a happy product (and a happy customer!).

Safety first! Before gracing store shelves, your creations need to navigate the world of regulations. Understanding labeling requirements, safety testing, and ingredient disclosures is essential. This ensures your brand not only thrives but also maintains a stellar reputation.

Ready to test the waters? Don't just take our word for it. Gather feedback through **market testing**. Give samples to a select group and see how their skin reacts. Listen to their thoughts on the scent, texture, and overall effectiveness. This valuable feedback allows you to refine your formulations and ensure your products are truly meeting consumer needs.

Branding is key! In a crowded market, you need to stand out. Craft a compelling story around the **unique benefits of bison tallow** and your commitment to **sustainable practices**. Utilize the power of social media, collaborate with influencers, and create educational content to spread the word about your brand and the magic of bison tallow.

Building your own bison tallow skincare line is an **ambitious adventure**. It requires creativity, a thirst for knowledge, and a dash of entrepreneurial spirit. By focusing on **quality, efficacy, and sustainability**, you have the potential to not only establish a thriving brand but also **positively impact the beauty industry and the environment**.

So, are you ready to turn your passion into a reality? This chapter equips you with the tools and knowledge to embark on this exciting journey. Remember, with dedication and a little bit of bison tallow magic, your skincare dreams can become a flourishing reality.

Chapter 6:
Bison Tallow: Nature's Fountain of Youth?

The quest for a youthful glow is as old as time itself. While modern science offers an array of solutions, sometimes the answer lies in ancient wisdom. Enter bison tallow, a **natural wonder** making waves in the beauty world. This chapter explores how bison tallow can be your secret weapon in the fight against aging and for **supercharged skin repair**.

Here's the secret: Bison tallow is a treasure trove of nutrients essential for keeping your skin **elastic and healthy**. Think of it as a multivitamin for your face! Vitamins A, D, E, and K work together like a well-oiled machine:

- **Vitamin A:** Picture this: your skin is constantly renewing itself. Vitamin A helps with that, promoting **cell regeneration**.
- **Vitamin D:** Think of it as sunshine for your skin, keeping it **healthy and strong**.
- **Vitamin E:** Imagine a shield protecting your skin from damage. Vitamin E acts as a powerful **antioxidant**, fighting off free radicals that can accelerate aging.

- **Vitamin K:** Ever scraped your knee and watched it heal? Vitamin K plays a similar role, aiding the skin's **healing process**.

The result? A complexion that's not just moisturized, but also **resilient** against the inevitable signs of aging.

But wait, there's more! Bison tallow mimics the natural oils our skin produces. This makes it an exceptional **moisturizer**, reinforcing our skin's **natural barrier**. Imagine a suit of armor protecting you from the elements. That's what this barrier does: keeping your skin hydrated and shielding it from pollutants and harsh UV rays – enemies of youthful skin.

Regular use of bison tallow-based products can be like giving your skin a **moisture makeover**. This translates to a **plumper, smoother appearance**, with less chance of fine lines and wrinkles stealing your shine.

Bonus tip: Bison tallow's **anti-inflammatory properties** come in handy for **skin repair**. Struggling with eczema, psoriasis, or dermatitis? Bison Tallow can help! By reducing inflammation, it promotes a **healthier healing process**, leading to improved texture and a diminished appearance of scars and marks.

Ready to ditch the harsh chemicals? Incorporating bison tallow into your routine can be a **game-changer** for anyone seeking natural anti-aging solutions. Whether you apply it directly or use formulated products, this natural wonder can **boost your skin's health** and leave you with a **radiant, youthful glow**.

Remember, true beauty comes from within, and sometimes, the answer lies in the wisdom of the past. Bison tallow is a testament to the power of nature's bounty, offering a **sustainable and effective** way to achieve lasting skin health and vitality.

Chapter 7:
Bison Tallow Hacks: Supercharge Your Daily Skincare Routine

Let's face it: our daily routines can get stuck in a rut. The same cleansers and moisturizers – it can all feel a bit...blah. But what if there was a natural ingredient that could **transform your skincare game**? Enter bison tallow, a **time-tested wonder** ready to **nourish and protect your skin** like never before.

This chapter dives into how to seamlessly integrate bison tallow into your **daily beauty regimen**, regardless of your skin type or concerns.

Morning Magic: Kickstart your day with a gentle cleanse. Follow it up with a **bison tallow-based moisturizer**. Here's the beauty: bison tallow mimics our natural oils, making it a **dreamy day cream**. It provides **lasting hydration** without clogging pores – perfect for all skin types!

Oily or acne-prone skin? Don't worry; we've got you covered. Look for formulations that combine bison tallow with **lightweight oils** that won't clog pores. Essential oils with **antibacterial properties** can be another bonus.

Nighttime Nourishment: After washing your face in the evening, apply a **bison tallow balm** to those dry patches or areas needing extra TLC. Remember, while you sleep, your skin goes into **repair mode**. Bison tallow's rich fatty acids **support this natural process**, promoting regeneration.

Want to take it up a notch? Look for products that blend bison tallow with superstars like **hyaluronic acid or retinol**. This combo can **boost the anti-aging effects**, leaving you with a youthful glow.

Treat Yourself: Spoil your skin with a weekly **bison tallow mask or serum**. These targeted treatments can address specific concerns, be it hydration, elasticity, or achieving a clearer complexion.

Mixing is key! Combine bison tallow with **clays, botanical extracts, or even gentle acids** to create powerful concoctions that leave your skin feeling **rejuvenated and radiant**.

Sensitive Skin? We hear you! Bison tallow's **soothing properties** can be a game-changer. Opt for **fragrance-free**

and chemical-free products. Look for formulations that combine the magic of bison tallow with calming ingredients like **chamomile or aloe vera**.

Remember, incorporating bison tallow isn't just about **glowing skin**. It's about embracing **sustainable and ethical practices**. Choose products that are **responsibly sourced and produced**. By doing so, you're not just treating your skin, and you're contributing to the **wellbeing of the environment** and supporting the revival of **ancient skincare wisdom**.

So, ditch the chemical-laden products and **embrace the power of nature**. Bison tallow is the key to a **healthy, radiant complexion** and a **guilt-free beauty routine**.

Chapter 8:

Hair Today, Gone Are the Bison Tallow Myths!

Ever wonder what your grandma used to get those long, luscious locks? Bison Tallow might just be the answer! This chapter tackles the common myths surrounding this **natural hair care hero** and reveals the **hair-raising benefits** it can offer.

Myth Buster #1: Greasy Hair Nightmare? Not a Chance!

Contrary to popular belief, using bison tallow the right way won't leave your hair looking like an oil slick. Here's the science: bison tallow is actually **compatible with your scalp's natural oils**. Think of it as a nourishing friend that conditions your hair without weighing it down. The key is to **use a little** and consider combining it with other natural goodies like oils to boost absorption and effectiveness.

Myth Buster #2: Not Just for the Dry-Haired Folks

Bison tallow is a **hair-type chameleon**. Its rich nutrient profile means it can benefit everyone, from those with dry, brittle strands to those prone to oily buildups. For oily hair, a little goes a long way. Bison tallow can help **regulate oil production**, leaving your hair feeling balanced. Dry or damaged hair? Bison tallow swoops in like a **deep conditioner**, bringing back its shine and health.

So, what makes bison tallow such a hair superstar? It's packed with vitamins and fatty acids that your hair craves. Vitamins A and E work their magic to **encourage growth and keep your scalp healthy**, while the fatty acids act as moisture magnets, **improving hair texture** and making it more manageable.

Here's the cherry on top: bison tallow's **antioxidant properties** shield your hair from environmental aggressors like pollution and UV rays – the ultimate defense against damage.

Ready to give your hair some TLC with bison tallow? It's easier than you think!

- **Pre-wash pampering:** Use a small amount as a **pre-shampoo treatment**.
- **DIY hair mask magic:** Mix it into your favorite homemade hair mask recipe for an extra nourishing boost.

- **Scalp SOS:** Melt a small amount of bison tallow and massage it into your scalp before washing. This can be a game-changer for dry scalps, reducing flakiness and promoting overall health.

Embracing bison tallow in your hair care routine is like stepping into a time machine where **ancient wisdom meets modern science**. As we rediscover the power of natural ingredients, bison tallow stands out as a **versatile and effective choice** for nurturing both your hair and skin. So, ditch the harsh chemicals and embrace the **natural way to healthy, happy hair!**

Chapter 9:

Honoring the Spirit of the Bison: A Legacy Woven into Native American Traditions

The mighty bison. Thundering across the plains, it's not just an animal – it's a symbol woven into the very fabric of Native American cultures. This chapter delves into the profound **respect and deep connection** these communities have shared with the bison for centuries.

Imagine a life deeply intertwined with nature. For countless Native American tribes, the bison wasn't just a source of sustenance; it represented **abundance, resilience, and the interconnectedness of all living things**. These majestic creatures provided for every need: food that nourished, clothing that protected, tools for daily life, and even shelter.

Respectful Harmony: The core principle guiding this relationship was one of **minimal waste and profound gratitude**. Every part of the bison was utilized, a testament to the deep understanding of the delicate balance within the ecosystem.

A Shadow Cast: Sadly, the 19th century witnessed a dark chapter. European settlers caused a drastic decline in bison populations, leaving a devastating impact on both the Native American way of life and the bison themselves.

A Time for Renewal: Thankfully, the story doesn't end there. Today, the **resurgence of bison herds** on Native American lands isn't just an ecological victory; it's a **cultural renaissance**. It signifies the revival of traditional practices and the rekindling of the ancient bond between humans and the bison.

Ethical Bison Tallow: Honoring the Legacy

This profound connection between Native American communities and the bison offers valuable lessons for the beauty industry, particularly in the use of bison tallow in cosmetic products.

Here's the key: **ethical sourcing**. Bison products should come from herds managed with **sustainability and respect** for both the animal and the land it roams.

By embracing these principles, the beauty industry can play a crucial role:

- **Conservation:** Supporting the revival of bison populations.
- **Cultural Heritage:** Acknowledging the significance of the bison in Native American traditions.

More than Just a Beauty Ingredient

This chapter compels us to look beyond the surface. Understanding the cultural and ethical significance of bison tallow adds a deeper layer of meaning to this ingredient. It encourages us to be **mindful and respectful** throughout the entire process, from sourcing to using bison-based beauty products.

So, the next time you hold a product containing bison tallow, remember the story it whispers. It's a tale of resilience, a testament to the enduring bond between humans and nature, and a call for a more **responsible and mindful approach** to the beauty products we choose.

Chapter 10:

Real People, Real Results: How Bison Tallow Transformed Their Skin

Forget celebrity endorsements; this chapter shines a light on the **real people** who have experienced the **remarkable effects** of incorporating Bison Tallow into their skincare routines.

Emily R.: From Flaky to Fantastic

"For years, my skin felt like the Sahara Desert - dry, itchy, and super sensitive. Harsh chemicals were out of the question. Then, a friend introduced me to bison tallow moisturizer. Let me tell you, I was **shocked**! My skin went from Sahara to **supple and glowy**. No more irritation, just **nourished, happy skin** that can finally keep up with my busy life."

John D.: Turning Back the Clock (Naturally!)

"Father Time was starting to show the wrinkles on my face. Is skin losing its bounce? Check. Feeling drier than a forgotten cactus? Absolutely. That's when I discovered a bison tallow-based skincare line. Now, my skin feels **firmer, smoother, and younger-looking**. Bonus points for the natural ingredients and the fact that they source their bison ethically. Sustainable skincare that actually works? Yes, please!"

Sarah L.: Battling Breakouts the Natural Way

"Acne breakouts were my constant companions. Trying every product under the sun, nothing seemed to work. I was wary of bison tallow, thinking it would clog my pores. But guess what? It did the complete opposite! My skin went from a battleground to **calm and clear**. Bison tallow somehow **balanced my oil production** and reduced inflammation. Who knew a natural solution could be so effective?"

Alex T.: Beauty with a Conscience

"When I learned about the sustainable practices and the deep cultural significance behind bison tallow, I knew I had to get on board. It's not just about what I put on my face; it's about the impact my choices have. And let me tell you, my skin is loving this switch! It's **healthy and glowing**, and I feel good knowing I'm **supporting ethical and eco-friendly practices**.

These are just a handful of the countless stories from people who have discovered the **power of bison tallow** for their skin. Their experiences highlight the importance of using **high-quality, ethically sourced ingredients**. They are a testament to the fact that **natural skincare solutions can truly transform your skin and your overall well-being**.

So, ditch the chemical-laden products and embrace the **natural path to healthy, radiant skin**. You might just be surprised by the results!

Chapter 11:
Bison Tallow: A Natural Beauty Revolution

The future of skincare is here, and it's being shaped by **ancient wisdom meeting modern innovation**. Buckle up, because bison tallow is about to become a **game-changer** in the beauty industry.

Nature's Treasure Trove: Bison tallow's versatility as an ingredient unlocks a treasure chest of possibilities for creating new and **effective skincare solutions**. Consumers are increasingly seeking **natural and sustainable products**, and Bison Tallow is perfectly positioned to answer this call.

Imagine a future where scientists unlock the full potential of bison tallow, combining it with other **powerful natural ingredients**. This paves the way for a new generation of skincare products that are **kind to your skin and kind to the planet**.

Beauty with a Conscience: Sustainability and ethical practices are no longer just buzzwords; they're becoming the norm. The good news? Bison Tallow aligns perfectly with this movement.

Thanks to successful conservation efforts and **sustainable farming practices**, bison populations are thriving. This ensures a **responsible source** for this unique ingredient. Bison tallow stands as a beacon of hope, proving that **beauty, environmental stewardship, and healthy skin** can go hand in hand.

Spreading the Knowledge: But this journey isn't just about science and ingredients. **Educating consumers** is key.

Imagine learning the fascinating story behind bison tallow, understanding its benefits, and appreciating the importance of **sustainable beauty practices**. Through compelling stories, **transparency** about sourcing, and fostering a **community around natural skincare**, brands can empower consumers to make informed choices and truly **appreciate the power of nature's bounty**.

A United Front: The future of bison tallow in the beauty industry isn't a solo act. It requires **collaboration** between various stakeholders.

Imagine a powerful alliance: indigenous communities sharing their knowledge, conservationists protecting bison populations, farmers ensuring ethical sourcing, and beauty brands working together. This collaboration ensures that using bison tallow **honors cultural heritage** promotes **ecological restoration**, and supports the economic well-being of communities involved in bison conservation.

Bison tallow's journey from a traditional remedy to a **cornerstone of modern natural beauty** is a testament to the industry's potential for positive change. Choosing bison tallow isn't just about incorporating a natural ingredient; it's about joining a **movement** toward a more **conscious, sustainable, and meaningful approach to beauty**.

So, the next time you reach for a skincare product, remember the story behind Bison Tallow. It's a story of tradition, innovation, and a future where **beauty and nature thrive in harmony**.

The Final Chapter:

Bison Tallow – Nature's Gift to Glowing Skin (and a Sustainable Future)

This book has been a whirlwind adventure, exploring the fascinating world of **bison tallow** - from its historical roots to its scientific potential as a **game-changer in the world of beauty**.

Remember that title: "The Bison Tallow Beauty Revolution"? It wasn't just catchy. Bison Tallow truly has the potential to **shake things up** in the skincare industry.

Why? Let's recap:

- **Nature's Powerhouse:** Bison tallow is packed with **nourishing fatty acids, vitamins, and antioxidants**. This translates to **deeply moisturized skin**, reduced inflammation, and a helping hand in **repairing and keeping wrinkles at bay**.
- **More Than Skin Deep:** Bison tallow isn't just about a pretty face. It carries the weight of **cultural significance** and **ethical sourcing**. Using it reminds us to be mindful of where our ingredients come from and the impact our choices

have on the environment and indigenous communities.

The revival of bison tallow is more than just a fad; it's a movement. A movement towards **natural, sustainable, and ethical beauty practices**.

Imagine a future where scientists unlock the full potential of bison tallow, creating innovative **skincare products that are kind to your skin and kind to the planet**.

The possibilities are endless:

- **Powerful new formulations:** Combining bison tallow with other natural wonders.
- **Sustainable sourcing practices:** Ensuring the well-being of bison herds and the communities involved.
- **A more informed consumer:** Making conscious choices about the products we use.

This isn't just about the beauty industry; it's a call to action for all of us.

We can be part of a **sustainable revolution**. We can support brands that prioritize **ethical sourcing** and

environmentally friendly practices. We can educate ourselves and spread the word about the **power of natural ingredients**.

This book is your **invitation to explore the possibilities**. It's a nudge to embrace **sustainable practices** and the revival of **traditional knowledge**. Remember, our skin, our communities, and our planet are all interconnected.

So, as we close this chapter, let's not just close the book. Let's **carry the inspiration forward**. Let's keep exploring the **rich tapestry of natural ingredients** that the world offers and use them to cultivate not just beautiful skin but a **more beautiful world**.

www.ingramcontent.com/pod-product-compliance
Lightning Source LLC
Chambersburg PA
CBHW051717250726
48653CB00008B/3077